Treasured Moments
Baby Journal

a beautiful, cheerful and adorable keepsake journal

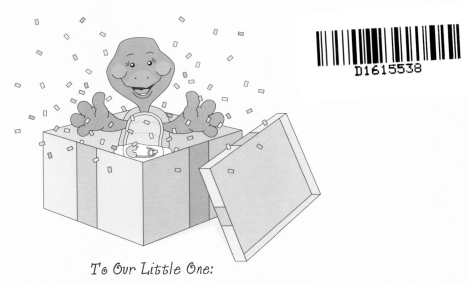

To Our Little One:

Thank you for making our wish come true.

"Of all nature's gifts to the human race,

what is sweeter than the gift of a child?"

~ *Marcus Tullius Cicer*

Treasured Moments

Baby Journal

a beautiful, cheerful and adorable keepsake journal

featuring

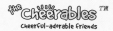

the Cheerables ™
cheerful-adorable friends

By Elizabeth & Alex Lluch

Published by Wedding Solutions Publishing, Inc.

Text copyright © 2005 by Wedding Solutions Publishing, Inc.

The Cheer-ables™ characters and illustrations are copyright © 2005 by Wedding Solutions Publishing, Inc.

poems by Sarah Jang

illustrated by David Defenbaugh

ISBN 1-887169-46-6

Printed in China

Table of Contents...

Newborn photo
page 19

Baby's first
steps
page 63

Baby's
homecoming
page 29

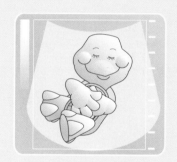

place photo here

Your Sonogram Photo

Before Your Arrival

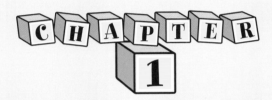

As minutes, hours and days go by,

time waiting for your birth seems to fly.

Preparing with joy for when you come our way,

we wait expectantly for this special day!

Daddy's side of the tree

Great Grandpa   Great Grandma   Great Grandpa   Great Grandma

Grandpa   Grandma

Daddy

Family

Mommy's side of the tree

_____   _____   _____   _____
Great Grandpa   Great Grandma   Great Grandpa   Great Grandma

_____   _____
Grandpa   Grandma

_____
Mommy

Tree

A mother's love...

Mommy's maiden name: _____

Birthday: _____

Hometown: _____ Height: _____

Color of hair: _____ Color of eyes: _____

Her favorite feature: _____

Favorite memories of her childhood: _____

_____

_____

What she hoped to be in the future: _____

_____

_____

Likes and dislikes: _____

_____

What she thought of daddy when they first met: _____

_____

"God cannot be everywhere, so he made mothers." ~ Arab proverb

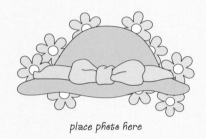

place photo here

Mommy Before You Were Born

A father's love...

Daddy's full name: _____

Birthday: _____

Hometown: _____ Height: _____

Color of hair: _____ Color of eyes: _____

His favorite feature: _____

Favorite memories of his childhood: _____

_____

_____

What he hoped to be in the future: _____

_____

_____

Likes and dislikes: _____

_____

What he thought of mommy when they first met: _____

_____

"The most important thing a father can do for his children is to love their mother." ~ Anon

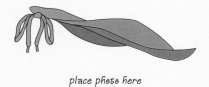

place photo here

Daddy Before You Were Born

A shower of love makes a baby grow...

When Baby Shower took place: _____

Where: _____

Host(s): _____

Theme: _____
_____

Who came to celebrate: _____
_____
_____

Special things we did to celebrate: _____
_____
_____

Gifts received: _____
_____
_____
_____

"I will send down showers in season; there will be showers of blessing."

~ Ezekiel 34:26

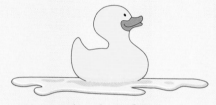

*place shower photo
or invitation here*

Your Baby Shower

Ready for your arrival...

How we chose your name: _____

_____

_____

What your name means: _____

_____

Your nickname: _____

Nursery color and theme: _____

_____

_____

What we did to get ready: _____

_____

_____

_____

Funny things that happened: _____

_____

"Three grand essentials to happiness in this life are something to do, something to love and something to hope for." ~ Joseph Addison

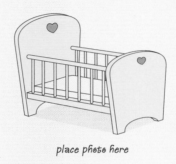

place photo here

Your Nursery

_____

_____

_____

_____

_____

_____

_____

_____

_____

_____

_____

_____

_____

_____ ~ _____

(signature and date)

"We find delight in the beauty and happiness of children that makes the heart too big for the body." ~ Ralph Waldo Emerson

The Arrival!

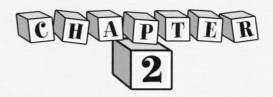

CHAPTER 2

Now is the time, today is the day.

Here comes the baby! Look! Make way!

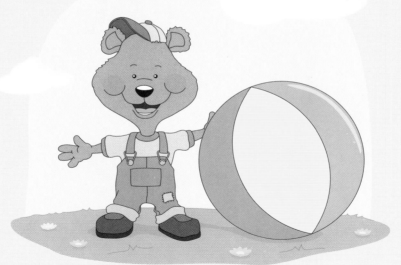

We give you our love, our special dear.

No more waiting... You're finally here!

Everything baby...

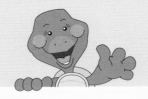

Birth date: _____

Time of delivery: _____

Location of hospital/delivery room: _____

Name of hospital/delivery room: _____

Mommy was in labor for: _____

Doctor/midwife's name: _____

People in the delivery room: _____

Who cut the umbilical cord: _____

Weight: _____

Length: _____

Color eyes: _____

Color hair: _____

Who you looked like: _____

How we celebrated your birth: _____

_____

_____

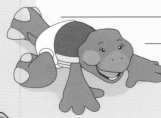

"Babies are such a nice way to start people." ~ Don Herold

The first to share our joy...

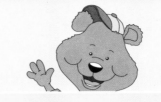
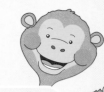

The first people to visit you: _____
_____
_____
_____

Who held you first: _____
_____
_____
_____

What they thought about you: _____
_____
_____
_____

Nice things they said: _____
_____

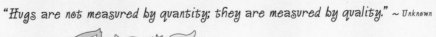

"Hugs are not measured by quantity; they are measured by quality." ~ Unknown

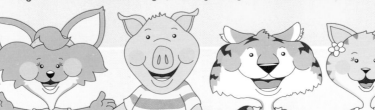

Chapter 2: The Arrival!

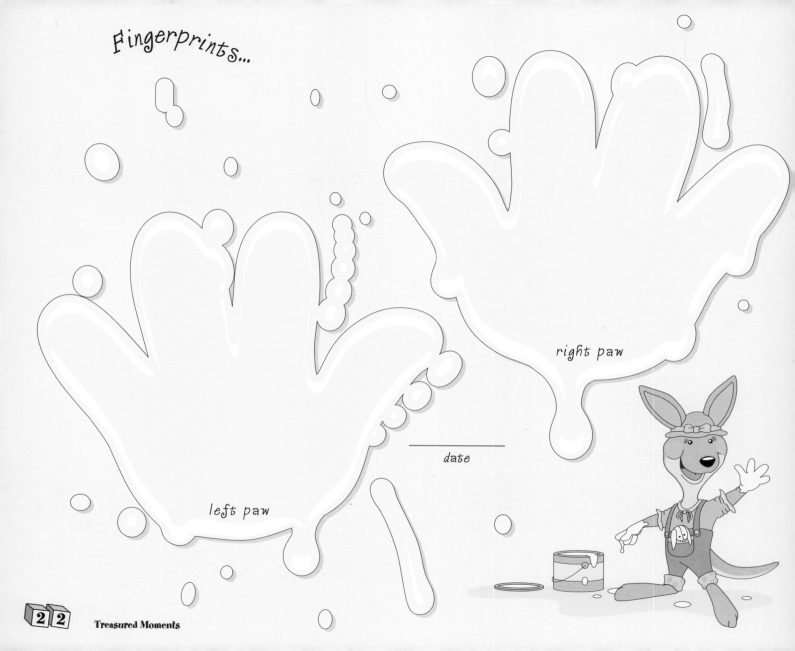

Fingerprints...

right paw

date

left paw

Treasured Moments

Footprints...

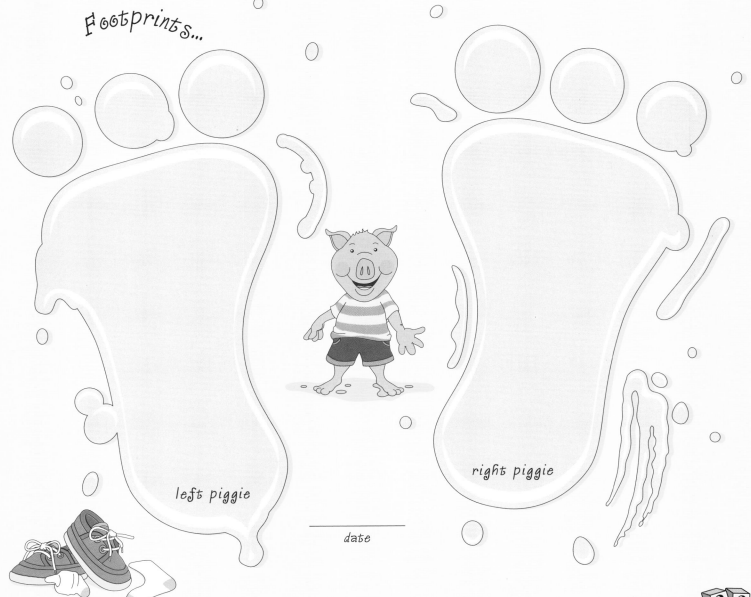

left piggie

right piggie

_____ date

Baby and Mommy...

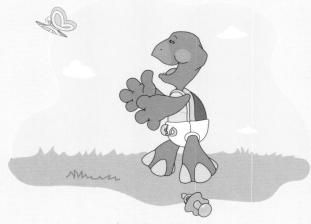

place photo of Mommy

holding baby here

You With Mommy

Baby and Daddy...

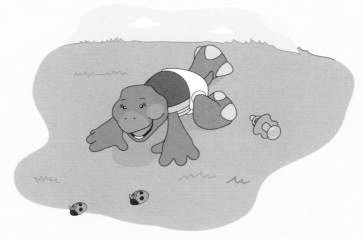

place photo of Daddy
holding baby here

You With Daddy

Reflections from the heart- the day you were born...

The Day Of Your Birth

_____

_____

_____

_____

_____

_____

_____

_____

_____

~ _____
(signature and date)

"A heart that loves is always young." ~ *Greek Proverb*

Your Homecoming

CHAPTER 3

Joyfully we bring you home,

a little baby to call our own.

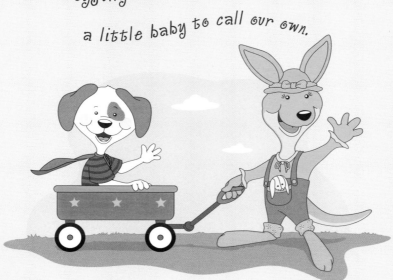

A bundle of joy, love, and laughter...

Here you will grow to live happily ever after!

No place like home...

Your first address: _____

How your siblings reacted: _____

_____

Who came to visit: _____

_____

What your visitors said about you: _____

_____

_____

Your temperament: _____

_____

How much you slept: _____

_____

How much you ate: _____

_____

"Our sweetest experiences of affection
are meant to point us to that realm which is
the real and endless home of the heart."
~ Henry Ward Beecher

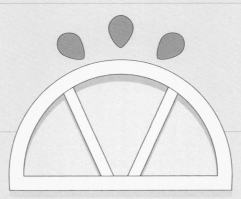

place "Homecoming" photo here

Your Homecoming

The world around you...

President of the United States: _____

Big news of the day: _____

_____

_____

_____

_____

Biggest toy fad: _____

_____

Popular movies: _____

_____

Hit songs: _____

_____

Musical groups: _____

_____

Television shows: _____

_____

"The sun does not shine for a few trees and flowers,
but for the wide world's joy." ~ Henry Ward Beecher

A whole new world...

Famous actors and actresses: _____

_____

Sports figures: _____

_____

Best-selling books: _____

_____

Fashion trends: _____

_____

_____

THE PRICE OF THINGS:

Gasoline: _____

Milk: _____

Diapers: _____

Postage stamp: _____

Other: _____

_____

"We all must work to make the world worthy of its children." ~ Pablo Casals

Presenting you to the world...

How we told the world: _____

_____

_____

_____

_____

_____

What the neighbors said: _____

_____

_____

How your pet(s) reacted: _____

_____

_____

Who bragged about you the most: _____

_____

_____

_____

"Little children are still the symbol of the eternal
marriage between love and duty." ~ George Eliot

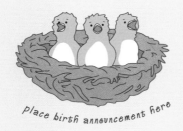

place birth announcement here

Your Birth Announcement

Good things come in small packages...

What you looked like: _____

_____

_____

How you like to be held: _____

_____

_____

What kind of sounds you made: _____

_____

_____

Nicknames after you were born: _____

_____

_____

_____

_____

"A very small degree of hope is sufficient to cause the birth of love."

~ Stendhal

Treasured Moments

Our bundle of joy...

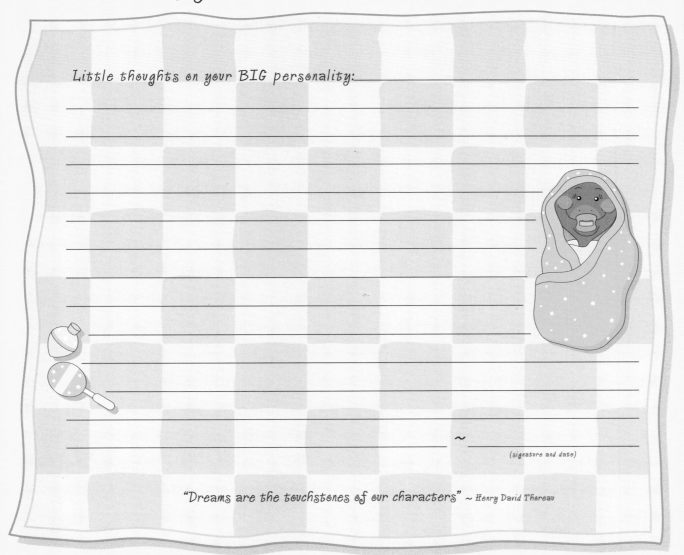

Little thoughts on your BIG personality: _____

_____

_____

_____

_____

_____

_____

_____

_____

_____

_____

~ _____
(signature and date)

"Dreams are the touchstones of our characters" ~ Henry David Thoreau

A reason to celebrate...

Christening, dedication, bris or special commemoration:

_____

_____

Date: _____

Where: _____

_____

What you wore: _____

_____

Who attended: _____

_____

_____

_____

Special gifts: _____

_____

_____

_____

"What better way to celebrate life than to have a child?"
~ Unknown

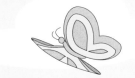

place photo of celebration here

Your Celebration

Reflections from the heart- enjoying your home...

_____   _____

_____

_____

_____

_____

_____

_____

_____

_____

_____

_____

_____

_____

_____

~ _____
(signature and date)

"Where we love is home,
home that our feet may leave,
but not our hearts."
~ Oliver Wendell Homes, Sr.

Treasured Moments

Your Favorite Things

CHAPTER 4

Kisses, hugs and butterflies...

Baby, love is in your eyes.

 We feel the joy each moment brings,

as you find your favorite things!

You just can't get enough of...

Favorite cuddle object: _____
_____

Favorite security object: _____
_____

Favorite song or lullaby: _____
_____

Favorite time to eat: _____
_____

Favorite time to sleep: _____
_____

Favorite person to hold you: _____
_____

Favorite way to be held: _____
_____

Other favorites: _____
_____

"Life is like jelly beans... And sometimes you get your favorite color." ~ Unknown

Your favorite things...

Favorite outfit: _____
_____

Favorite place to visit: _____
_____

Favorite thing to do: _____
_____

Favorite book: _____
_____

Favorite pet: _____
_____

Favorite friends: _____
_____

Favorite games: _____
_____

Other favorites: _____
_____

"A mind once stretched by a new idea never regains its original dimension."
~ Oliver Wendell Holmes, Sr.

Wagging tails and happy faces...

Pretty songs and warm embraces.

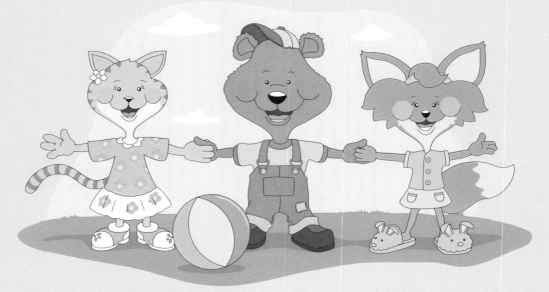

Making memories of joy with each other,

as you find things that you love like no other!

"Joyfulness keeps the heart young."
~ Orison Swett Marden

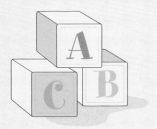

place photo of baby with

favorite toy here

Your Favorite Toy

Grandparents... your favorite kind of love - unconditional

Mommy's parents: _____

Their loving thoughts about you: _____

_____

_____

_____

Daddy's parents: _____

Their loving thoughts about you: _____

_____

_____

_____

Great-grandparents: _____

Family traditions: _____

_____

_____

_____

_____

"Grandmas and Grandpas are just like moms and dads,
but with more frosting." ~ Unknown

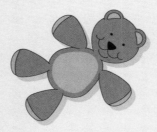

place photo of baby with

grandparents here

Your Grandparents

Nothing says "love" more than family...

Your Aunts and Uncles: _____

_____

Their loving thoughts about you: _____

_____

_____

Cousins: _____

Their loving thoughts about you: _____

_____

_____

Favorite family stories: _____

_____

_____

_____

_____

_____

"Families are like fudge... Mostly sweet with a few nuts." ~ Unknown

4 6   **Treasured Moments**

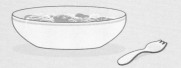

place photo of baby with relatives here

Your Relatives

_____

_____

_____

_____

_____

_____

_____

_____

_____

_____

_____

_____

~ _____

(signature and date)

"A thankful heart is not only the greatest virtue, but the parent of all other virtues."

~ Marcus Tullius Cicero

Look At You Grow!

Your First Year

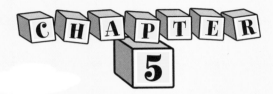

Bigger and better, day by day,

we see you now in every way.

Laughing, smiling as you go...

We watch you as you grow and grow!

Your baby days go by so fast...

MONTH ONE:

    Date: _____   Weight: _____   Length: _____

    Comments: _____

MONTH TWO:

    Date: _____   Weight: _____   Length: _____

    Comments: _____

MONTH THREE:

    Date: _____   Weight: _____   Length: _____

    Comments: _____

MONTH FOUR:

    Date: _____   Weight: _____   Length: _____

    Comments: _____

MONTH FIVE:

    Date: _____   Weight: _____   Length: _____

    Comments: _____

MONTH SIX:

    Date: _____   Weight: _____   Length: _____

    Comments: _____

"If you want 1 year of prosperity, grow grain. If you want 10 years of prosperity, grow trees.
If you want 100 years of prosperity, grow babies." ~ Chinese Proverb

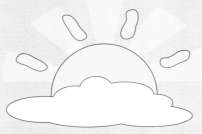

place photo of baby between the

ages of 1-6 months here

You At Age 1-6 Months

Soon diapers will be in your past...

MONTH SEVEN:

    Date: _____   Weight: _____   Length: _____

    Comments: _____

MONTH EIGHT:

    Date: _____   Weight: _____   Length: _____

    Comments: _____

MONTH NINE:

    Date: _____   Weight: _____   Length: _____

    Comments: _____

MONTH TEN:

    Date: _____   Weight: _____   Length: _____

    Comments: _____

MONTH ELEVEN:

    Date: _____   Weight: _____   Length: _____

    Comments: _____

MONTH TWELVE:

    Date: _____   Weight: _____   Length: _____

    Comments: _____

"A baby is born with a need to be loved- and never outgrows it."
~ Frank A. Clark

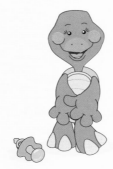

place photo of baby between the

ages of 7-12 months here

You At Age 7-12 Months

Reflections from the heart- how fast you've grown...

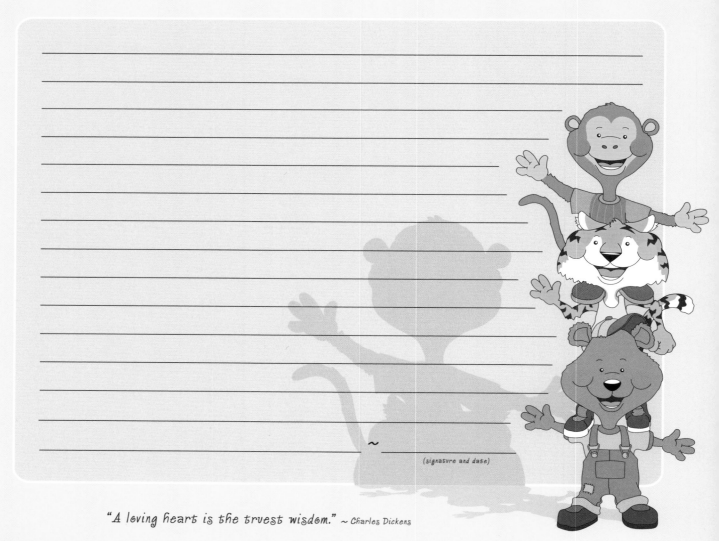

_____

_____

_____

_____

_____

_____

_____

_____

_____

_____

_____

~ _____
(signature and date)

"A loving heart is the truest wisdom." ~ Charles Dickens

There's A First Time For Everything!

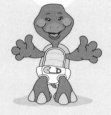

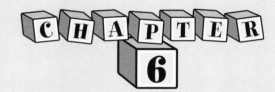

CHAPTER 6

I can't believe you've come so far.

You're quickly becoming who you are.

A bath, a step, a word you speak...

Each new first makes you unique!

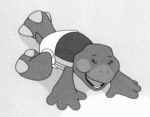

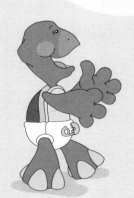

The first step...

Personality- The first time you...

    Smiled: _____

    Laughed: _____

    Waved bye-bye: _____

    Played peek-a-boo: _____

Habits- The first time you...

    Slept through the night: _____

    Bathed in a bathtub: _____

    Went potty: _____

    Stopped wearing diapers: _____

    Dressed yourself: _____

Chatterbox- The first time you...

    Said your first word: _____

    Said ABC's: _____

    Sang a song: _____

"The beginning of wisdom is calling things
by their right names." ~ Chinese Proverb

It's only the beginning...

Actions- The first time you...

Held your head up: _____

Rolled over: _____

Scooted or crawled: _____

Sat up: _____

Food- The first time you...

Held a bottle: _____

Ate baby food: _____

Ate solid food: _____

Fed yourself: _____

Around and About- The first time you...

Danced: _____

Drew a picture: _____

Made a friend: _____

Took a trip: _____

Other firsts: _____

"What we call results are beginnings." ~ Ralph Waldo Emerson

The very first time you got a haircut...

When: _____

Where: _____

Cost: _____

Who cut your hair: _____

What other people thought: _____

_____

_____

_____

How you reacted: _____

_____

_____

_____

_____

"Love is a great beautifier." ~ Louisa May Alcott

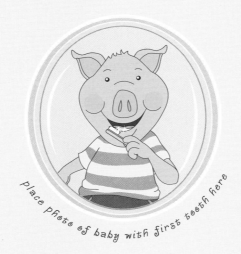

place photo of baby with first tooth here

Your First Tooth

Baby steps...

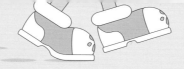

The First Time You:

Pulled yourself up to standing: _____

Stood on your own: _____

Took your first steps: _____

What we did to celebrate your accomplishment: _____

_____

_____

_____

_____

Funny stories about your first steps: _____

_____

_____

_____

_____

_____

_____

"Our greatest glory is not in never falling, but in rising every time we fall."

~ Confucius

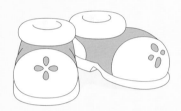

place photo of baby's
first steps here

Your First Steps

Your very first sleepover...

When: _____

Where we went: _____
_____

What we packed in your diaper bag: _____
_____

What we did: _____
_____

Who we saw while we were out: _____
_____

What they said about you: _____
_____
_____

What you thought about the outside world: _____
_____
_____
_____

"What we have to learn to do, we learn by doing." ~ Aristotle

Your very first trip...

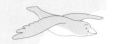

When: _____

Where we went: _____

_____

How we got there: _____

_____

_____

Couldn't leave home without: _____

_____

_____

What you thought about traveling: _____

_____

_____

_____

_____

_____

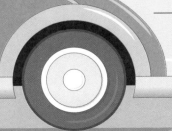

"The world is a book, and those who do not travel read only one page."

~ Saint Augustine

Chapter 6: There's a First Time For Everything!

Your very first holidays...

Holiday: _____ Date: _____

What we did to celebrate: _____

_____

_____

_____

Holiday: _____ Date: _____

What we did to celebrate: _____

_____

_____

_____

Holiday: _____ Date: _____

What we did to celebrate: _____

_____

_____

_____

"The most effective kind of education is that a child should play amongst lovely things."

~ Plato

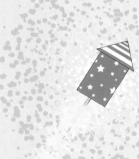

place photo of baby

celebrating a holiday here

Your Holiday Celebration

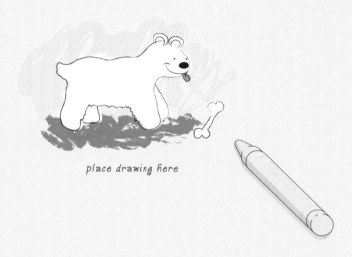

place drawing here

Your First Drawing

It's your very first pet...

Your first pet was a: _____

Pet's name: _____

What you thought about your pet: _____

_____

_____

_____

What your pet thought about you: _____

_____

_____

How you got along together: _____

_____

_____

_____

_____

_____

_____

home

"The dog was created especially for children. He is the God of frolic."

~ Henry Ward Beecher

Reflections from the heart- a time for firsts...

_____

_____

_____

_____

_____

_____

_____

_____

_____

_____

_____

_____ ~ _____
(signature and date)

"Where your pleasure is, there is your treasure: where your treasure,
there your heart; where your heart, there your happiness."
~ Saint Augustine

Treasured Moments

Happy First Birthday!

CHAPTER 7

Oh my gosh, you're one year old!

12 months together, to have and to hold.

A wonderful year we've shared with eachother...

Had so much fun, we can't wait for another!

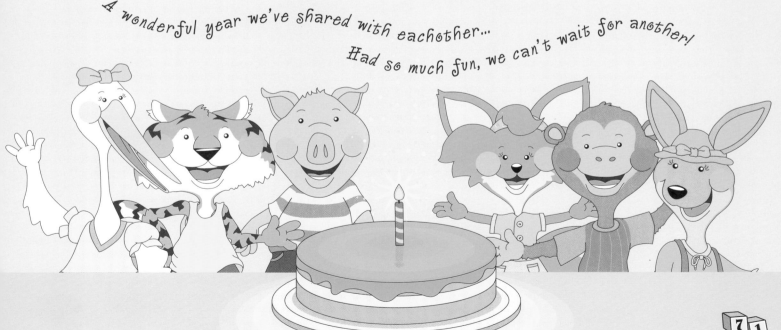

Your first birthday celebration...

Theme of your party: _____

What made your party special: _____
_____

Your cake was: _____

What you did with the cake: _____
_____

Who helped you celebrate:

_____

_____

_____

_____

_____

_____

Gifts:

_____

_____

_____

_____

_____

_____

"You have to eat the first piece of candy before you can eat the whole bag." ~ Unknown

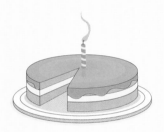

place photo of baby

celebrating first birthday here

Your First Birthday Party

All about your first year...

Height: _____

Weight: _____

How you looked: _____

_____

Your personality: _____

_____

You enjoyed saying things like: _____

_____

Things you've learned to do this year: _____

_____

The most memorable moment this year: _____

_____

_____

_____

_____

"The spirit of youth never grows old." ~ Unknown

Your favorites at one year...

Foods to eat: _____
_____

Books to read: _____
_____

Activities: _____
_____

Toys to play with: _____
_____

Clothes to wear: _____
_____

People to be with: _____
_____

Things to do: _____
_____

More favorites: _____

"What is a friend? A single soul dwelling in two bodies." ~ Aristotle

One-year old likes and dislikes...

Things you really liked:_____

_____

_____

Things you really did not like: _____

_____

_____

Funny stories that happened this year: _____

_____

_____

_____

_____

_____

_____

"I've learned that you can't hide a piece of broccoli in a glass of milk." ~ Child Age 7

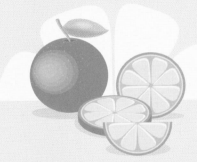

place photo of baby at
one year old here

You At Age 1

 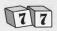

_____

_____

_____

_____

_____

_____

_____

_____

_____

_____

_____

_____ ~ _____
(signature and date)

"What comes from the heart goes to the heart." ~ Samuel Taylor Coleridge

A Year Anew... Now You're Two!

CHAPTER 8

Two years have past with joy and cheer,
we can't believe your birthday is here.

Two years of laughs and hugs and grins...
Can't wait to see what next year brings!

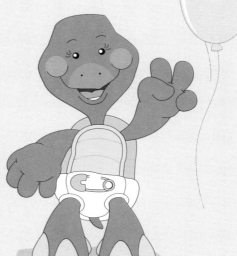

Your second birthday celebration...

Theme of your party: _____

What made your party special: _____
_____

Your cake was: _____

What you did with the cake: _____
_____

Who helped you celebrate: Gifts:

_____   _____

_____   _____

_____   _____

_____   _____

_____   _____

_____   _____

_____   _____

_____   _____

"One must ask children and birds how cherries and strawberries taste."
~ Johann Wolfgang von Goethe

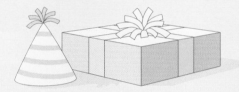

place photo of baby
celebrating second birthday here

Your Second Birthday Party

All about your second year...

Height: _____

Weight: _____

How you looked: _____

_____

Your personality: _____

_____

You enjoyed saying things like: _____

_____

Things you've learned to do this year: _____

_____

The most memorable moment this year: _____

_____

_____

_____

_____

"We are most nearly ourselves when we
achieve the seriousness of the child at play." ~ Heraclitus

Your favorites at two years...

Foods to eat: _____
_____

Books to read: _____
_____

Activities: _____
_____

Toys to play with: _____
_____

Clothes to wear: _____
_____

People to be with: _____
_____

Things to do: _____
_____

More favorites: _____

"To be in your child's memories tomorrow,
be in his or her life today." ~ Unknown

Little person... big opinions...

Things you really liked: _____
_____
_____

Things you really did not like: _____
_____
_____

Funny stories that happened this year: _____
_____
_____
_____
_____
_____
_____
_____

"A baby is God's opinion that life should go on."
~ Carl Sandburg

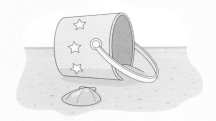

place photo of baby at
2 years old here

You At Age 2

Reflections from the heart- your second year...

_____

_____

_____

_____

_____

_____

_____

_____

_____

_____

_____   ~ _____

                                                                  (signature and date)

"...May your heart be filled with gladness

to cheer you." ~ Irish blessing

Say "Hooray!" You're Three Today!

CHAPTER 9

Who knew time could move so fast?

In just a wink, you're three at last.

Taller, smarter, bigger, stronger...

Baby days are here no longer!

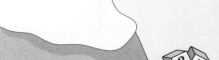

Your third birthday celebration...

Theme of your party: _____

What made your party special: _____
_____

Your cake was: _____

What you did with the cake: _____
_____

Who helped you celebrate: Gifts:

_____   _____

_____   _____

_____   _____

_____   _____

_____   _____

_____   _____

_____   _____

"All good things which exist are the fruits of originality." ~ John Stuart Mill

Treasured Moments

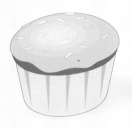

place photo of baby

celebrating third birthday here

Your Third Birthday Party

All about your third year...

Your height: _____

Your weight: _____

How you looked: _____

_____

Your personality: _____

_____

You enjoyed saying things like: _____

_____

Things you've learned to do this year: _____

_____

The most memorable moment this year: _____

_____

_____

_____

_____

"Of all the music that reached farthest into heaven,
is the beating of a loving heart" ~Henry Ward Beecher

Treasured Moments

Your favorites at three years...

Foods to eat: _____

_____

Books to read: _____

_____

Activities: _____

_____

Toys to play with: _____

_____

Clothes to wear: _____

_____

People to be with: _____

_____

Things to do: _____

_____

More favorites: _____

_____

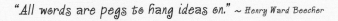

"All words are pegs to hang ideas on." ~ Henry Ward Beecher

Chapter 9: Say "Hooray!" You're Three Today!

The third time's a charm...

Things you really liked: _____

_____

_____

Things you really did not like: _____

_____

_____

Funny stories that happened this year: _____

_____

_____

_____

_____

_____

_____

_____

"Better keep yourself clean and bright: you are the window through which you must see the world." ~ Sir Walter Besant

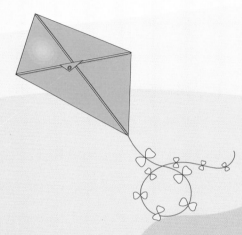

place photo of baby
at 3 years old here

You At Age 3

Reflections from the heart- your third year...

_____

_____

_____

_____

_____

_____

_____

_____

_____

_____

_____

_____ ~ _____

(signature and date)

"Fill your heart with good things, and good things
will follow you for the rest of your life." ~ Unknown

Your Future Is Bright!

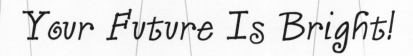

A hope, a wish, upon a star...

These past three years, we've come so far.

Our love and support we give to you,

and wish the best in all you do!

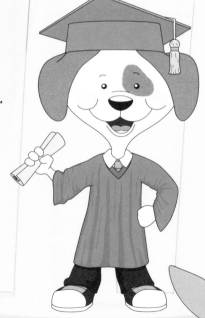

Reflections from the heart- your future...

From Mommy: _____
_____
_____
_____
_____
_____
_____
_____
_____
_____
_____
_____
_____ ~ _____
                              (signature and date)

"Who takes the child by the hand takes the mother by the heart."
~ German Proverb

Treasured Moments

Reflections from the heart- your future...

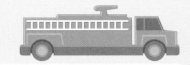

From Daddy: _____

_____

_____

_____

_____

_____

_____

_____

_____

_____

_____

_____

~ _____

(signature and date)

"A father's heart lies in his child's hopes." ~ Unknown

Your Star Shines Bright!

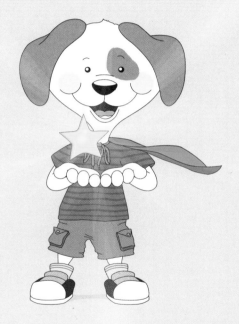

"Go confidently in the direction of your dreams. Live the life you have imagined."
~ Henry David Thoreau